Coils & Curls
The Hair Product Handbook

Helping the Product Junkies of the world
buy **SMARTER**, sort through marketing
HYPE and save **MONEY!**

Nicole Harmon

CONTENTS

This book is dedicated to every woman who has ever struggled with her hair.

And to my husband John, for loving and supporting me enough to help my dreams become reality.

Introduction

The Hair Liberty Story

I got my first kiddie perm at the age of 8. As soon as my mom said my hair was done, I went straight to the bathroom, put a little water on a brush and ran it through my hair. Needless to say, my mom was very upset. She couldn't understand why I ruined all of her hard work. That was a long time ago, but I still remember my 8-year old reasoning. Surely, after all that time she spent doing this "treatment", my hair would be "easy". After all those hours, I was sure that my hair would be just like all the other girls at school. I wouldn't have to run from the rain or wear a shower cap in the bathtub. I didn't have to fear water because my hair was "fixed".

Of course, I was oh so wrong. My hair still seemed to be a burden...a big ball of cotton that never looked anything like my doll's hair. People called my hair "nappy", "a mess", and "too much work", so I spent 10 years with it hidden in braids and cornrows. I was happy for a while because my hair was "under control" and I didn't really have to deal with it. But, by the time I finished my first year at college, I was fed up with wearing braids. I decided to spend some of the money I earned working on campus to get a relaxer.

The relaxer brought me joy and what initially seemed like freedom. I could finally do my own hair! I washed and blow dried it every few days and religiously went to the salon for touch ups every 5 weeks. I always got compliments on looking polished and put together (even during 8 am classes). Sadly, that freedom didn't last long. My hair seemed to stop growing and I noticed breakage with every stroke of the comb. I was doing my hair just like they did it at the salon, and my bathroom cabinet was filled with products, but something was still wrong. So, you know what comes next...weaves, glorious weaves! It started with a few tracks and escalated to a full sew-in. Talk about easy, right? I finally had long, soft hair that looked great even if I didn't do much with it. I was content, but still unsatisfied. What was wrong with MY hair?

In the spring of 2003, I graduated from college wearing a full sew-in. At the same time, unbeknownst to me, the hair care industry was going through a major shift. As I was starting my weave binge, Mahisha Dellinger debuted her line of products called CURLS and Shelley Davis launched Kinky-Curly Hair Products. Soon after that, Pantene rolled out the Relaxed & Natural Collection and Titi and Miko Branch launched Miss Jessie's Natural Hair Products. For the first time, our natural hair was being described as curly and coily instead of frizzy and nappy. Entrepreneurs and big product manufacturers began competing for our hair care dollars by making products that could actually deliver strength and moisture for our dry, fragile strands. It was like an Ethnic Hair Care Renaissance, and it's actually still happening today. New and better products come out every year as

companies listen to our feedback and step up their game.
However, back in 2003, I had no idea that was all happening. I was
still spending most of my extra time and money to maintain my
hair at the salon and I didn't know there was another way.

Everything changed when I was about to deep condition
one day in 2009. I was trying to revive my hair after three nonstop
years of weaves. Instead of plopping on the conditioner and
sitting under the dryer, I decided to read the directions for once.
To my surprise, the instructions on the product didn't mention
anything about applying heat. Why hadn't I ever noticed that
before? I knew after years of effort that sitting under the dryer
hadn't solved my hair problems, so why did I continue to do it? By
this point, I was pursuing a degree in Pharmacy and for the first
time I realized that the chemistry I was studying in college actually
applied to hair products. I started wondering what was different
about products that required heat. As I began exploring hair care
ingredients, I discovered that cosmetic scientists and
dermatologists had been studying hair of African descent for
almost 2 decades!

I learned to look for the right terms as I continued my
cosmetic chemistry research. You won't find the word "nappy" in
scientific journals, but you will find the words "tightly coiled" and
"overly porous". I obsessively researched hair care science and
cosmetic chemistry to compare what I was learning to the trials
and triumphs women were sharing in the burgeoning natural hair

community online. In 2010, I launched HairLiberty.org, a website dedicated to science-based ethnic hair care information. The following year, I made the big decision to change careers from pharmaceutical science to cosmetic chemistry and soon after that I was admitted to the Society of Cosmetic Chemists. All of my research over the past 3 years comes down to this: **Your product choices and styling techniques will determine if you love or hate your hair.** That's true for everyone, but it's exceptionally true for women with coils and curls. The challenge these days is to find the perfect combination of products and techniques that will help you style your hair exactly the way you want it. It doesn't matter how kinky or dry your strands may be, whether you love springy coils or a sleek bob, there are dozens of great products that will fit your needs.

Use this handbook to learn how to sort through the hype and pinpoint products that will moisturize, strengthen, and smooth your coils and curls. Commit to practicing a routine that delivers the results you want, so you can have the freedom to rock any style your heart desires. Curly, straight, natural, relaxed, whatever! That's what I call Hair Liberty and it's time to free yourself!

Know the Hair You Have to Get the Hair You Want

Dry, Curly, Coily, Coarse, Fine, Chemically-Treated, Frizzy, Weak, Color-treated...

Product labels are filled with descriptive words. Knowing which ones apply to your hair will help you choose products that can deliver the results you want.

Terms to Know

Let's make sure we're speaking the same language

Hair products promise all kinds of things from faster hair growth to thicker strands. There are a few terms you need to know before we can start sorting through the hype.

Follicle – The hair follicle is the only "living" part of your hair. Each follicle is embedded in your scalp and connected to your blood supply. A hair product that promises increased hair growth will need to be applied to your scalp and hair follicles for at least 2 minutes in order to be effective. The size of each follicle determines the size of the strand of hair that grows out of it.

Cortex – The cortex is the inner core of each strand of hair. Think of it like the inside of a tree trunk. A product that promises to deep condition your hair will not deliver results unless it contains water and other ingredients that can absorb into the cortex. Scientific research shows that hair of African descent typically has lower levels of moisture in the cortex than other hair types.

Cuticle – If the cortex of each strand is like a tree trunk, the cuticles are like layers of tree bark. Each cuticle layer is stacked on top of the next to protect the cortex. The cuticle makes up the surface of each strand, which means it is the most easily damaged part of your hair. The kinks (bends) on coily strands only start out with one or two cuticle layers, compared to 5 to 10 layers on other parts of the hair; so by definition coils are more prone to damage than other hair types. The cuticles of curly and coily hair are also more likely to be ruffled and lifted from basic combing and styling. Most hair products are designed to resurface and smooth the cuticle.

Porosity – Hair and skin are porous which means they can absorb water and other ingredients. The "gap in coverage" caused by the lifted and ruffled cuticles on coily hair allows the cortex to lose moisture almost as quickly as it is absorbed, leaving the hair overly porous. All hair types become more porous the longer the hair gets and there is no permanent fix for high porosity (no matter what a product claims). The only remedies are to re-moisturize the hair often and to use products that can partially patch the cuticle. It is also important to get the hair trimmed periodically to remove the oldest, most porous ends.

Substantive – In order for your rinse out products to deliver lasting results, they have to contain ingredients that are "substantive". Substantive ingredients are so strongly attracted to the protein in your hair that they can overcome the force of the water and stay attached to your strands after you do your final rinse. In order to keep your hair smooth and manageable between washes, it is important to choose products that are filled with "substantive" ingredients. The most important substantive ingredients for coily and curly hair are cationic conditioners and hydrolyzed protein. You will learn more about those ingredients in Chapter 2. Pure oils and butters are not usually substantive to the hair so it is best to save those for your leave-in products.

Top 5 – Hair product ingredients are usually listed in descending order. The ingredient in the highest amount is usually listed first, and the ingredient in the lowest amount is last. When you see a reference to the "top 5", I am referring to the first five ingredients on the product label. Some ingredients do not have to be in the top 5 to be effective. (If you listed the ingredients of a cake, baking powder would not be in the top 5, but it's still important.) Use the top 5 as your starting point as you begin deciphering product labels.

Curl Types

Coils & Curls by the Numbers

Years ago, Andre Walker (Oprah's hair stylist of over 2 decades) published a system to categorize different hair textures. His "curl typing" system is a great place to start when you begin learning about your coils and curls. But that's all it is, a place to start...and keep it movin! You won't see curl types mentioned in this book very often because I don't want you to get caught up in trying to categorize your hair. The most important thing to know about coils and curls aka "Curl Types 3 and 4" is that they have a higher risk of breakage and dryness. Type 4 is the most breakage prone of all hair types because the strands are not just curly, they are coily. Hair that is "coily" has tight twists and turns that make it weaker and more likely to break whenever it is combed.

It seems like knowing your curl type could help you determine how to care for your hair (how often to wash, which products to use, etc.) but that is not the case. In my opinion, your curl type has more to do with styling than maintenance. See, if you have "Type 4" coils and you prefer a sleek Toni Braxton-style cut, you need to realize that is a Type 1 style. This is about Hair Liberty so please believe you are free to rock that look! However, when you style "against type", it is important to follow a consistent regimen that allows you to get the look you want without sacrificing your hair. The further your desired style is from your natural texture, the more attention you will need to pay to your product choices and styling techniques. Always keep that in mind as you choose your go-to hairstyles.

Type 1 – Straight Hair
Breakage Risk: Lowest
Porosity: Lowest

Type 3 – Curly Hair
Breakage Risk: Medium
Porosity: Medium to High

Type 2 – Wavy Hair
Breakage Risk: Low
Porosity: Low to Medium

Type 4 – Coily Hair
Breakage Risk: Highest
Porosity: Highest

②

Read Hair Product Labels

Like an Expert

The descriptions and ingredients on the label will tell you if a product is a good match for your hair. You just have to know what to look for!

Hair Product Basics

Whether your coils and curls are natural or relaxed, I think we can all agree that we want smooth, manageable hair. Please let go of any ideas that the "quality" of your hair is determined by genetics. **Your product choices and styling techniques will determine whether you love or hate your hair.** If you do not like the way your hair looks, it is simply time to start a new routine. Think of your hair like your face, when you wake up looking tired and dull, you don't just go out like that. You wash, moisturize, and maybe put on some makeup. You can and should do the same things for your hair (switch the makeup for a leave-in or two). Just like with your skin, when you find the right product matches, everything else gets easier.

You will find the best products for your hair by reading the labels. Not just the front of the bottle that uses hyped up words like "nourishing", "replenishing", and "restoring", but the back of the bottle where the ingredients are listed. We will go over the key ingredients you need to look for, product by product in this chapter.

As you read this chapter, keep a few things in mind:

• Hair products deliver temporary, not permanent results. Even when a product promises to "repair" or "restore" it really means with continued use. The effects of most products will only last until you wash your hair again. The best products contain substantive ingredients that will keep your hair smooth and manageable for up to 3 washes at a time.

• Always use rinse-out products according to the instructions on the container. Many hair products, even if they are labeled "natural" or "organic", contain ingredients that should not be left in contact with your skin for long periods. The best way to limit negative health effects from cosmetic products is to use them as directed. There's more info about safety at the end of this chapter.

• Don't be appeased by soft hair. It is easy to make your hair soft. It is not easy to make it smoother and less breakage prone. Make sure your staple products have the key ingredients outlined in this section, or they are probably not worth your money.

Find the Best Shampoos

First things first, you NEED a good shampoo in your life! A good shampoo keeps your scalp healthy (which means better hair growth) and makes your hair easier to comb. A bad shampoo will lead to drier hair, scalp irritation, and unstoppable frizz. Your shampoo is truly the first step to smooth, manageable coils and curls.

The best shampoos contain:

• Sulfate-free detergents to prevent excessive dryness and scalp irritation
• Cationic ingredients to condition your hair while you cleanse
• pH adjusters to balance the pH of the shampoo and prevent unnecessary cuticle damage while you wash

Sulfate-free Detergents

Have you noticed all the sulfate-free shampoos popping up? It sounds like classic marketing hype, but there are a few good reasons to avoid sulfate detergents. Every cleansing product, whether it is shampoo or laundry detergent, contains surfactants (pronounced sir•fac•tents). Surfactants are the ingredients that allow oil to be dissolved from a dirty surface. If you ever put dish soap on a pot and leave it to soak, you are waiting for the surfactants in your dish soap to break up the grease left from your food. Surfactants made with sulfates like sodium lauryl sulfate and sodium laureth sulfate have been used in shampoo for many years, but current scientific research has found them to be significantly irritating for the scalp and drying to the hair.

Does that mean your hair will drastically improve if you start using a "sulfate-free shampoo"? Maybe not. Most women are using sulfate-based shampoos because that is the majority of what's on the market. Even if a shampoo contains sulfates, it can still be formulated to work well for your hair. Cosmetic scientists often combine sulfates with gentler surfactants to create a mild, but effective product. However, I want you to have the most up to date information and the fact is sulfate-based shampoos are not the best way to cleanse our naturally dry strands.

To find the gentlest shampoos, look for products that contain at least one of the surfactants listed below.

Gentle surfactants to look for in your shampoo:
Coco-Glucoside
Decyl Glucoside
Disodium Cocoamphodipropionate
Disodium Laureth Sulfosuccinate

Disodium Lauroamphodiacetate

Sodium Cocoyl Isethionate

Sodium Methyl Cocoyl Taurate

Harsh/Drying surfactants to skip:

Sodium Laureth Sulfate

Sodium Lauryl Sulfate

Ammonium Lauryl Sulfate

Ammonium Laureth Sulfate

Sodium Myreth Sulfate

Saponified Oils*

Soap*

Visit HairLiberty.org to learn why it's best to avoid washing your hair with soap and saponified oils.

Cationic Conditioners

It is best to choose products that condition your hair at every step of your routine...during cleansing, after cleansing, and before styling. It probably seems like shampoo cannot cleanse and condition at the same time, but cosmetic chemistry makes it possible. You know how clothes get stuck together in the dryer and they make a popping sound when you pull them apart? That happens because of something called static charge. Coils and curls often have a negative ionic charge that causes constant frizz and fly aways. You can make your hair smoother and easier to comb by choosing a shampoo that contains positively charged conditioning ingredients called "cationics". The ingredients listed below spread over your hair while you lather the shampoo and they stay locked to your strands while dirt and product residue rinse away (that means cationics are substantive ingredients). The cationic ingredients deposited on your hair by your shampoo will also help you detangle once the conditioner is in.

Cationic Conditioners to look for in your shampoo:
Amodimethicone
Cassia Hydroxypropyltrimonium Chloride
Guar Hydroxypropyltrimonium Chloride
Polyquaternium-7
Polyquaternium-10
Polyquaternium-11
Polyquaternium-44
Polyquaternium-47

pH Adjusters

The pH value of a liquid tells you whether it is an acid (like orange juice) or a base (like baking soda mixed with water). pH values below 7 are acids, values above 7 are called bases. Skin and hair are made of keratin proteins and all types of protein are sensitive to pH. Our skin and hair can better maintain their natural strength when they are kept at acidic pH values between 4.5 and 6.5 during cleansing. Manufacturers do not make shampoos with pH values below 4, but there are a few shampoos out there above pH 7. When the shampoo is basic instead of acidic, the outer cuticle of your hair will swell and lift excessively when you lather up. When your hair dries later, you will be left with the kind of volume you don't like...stubborn frizz and tangles. Shampoos that are pH balanced help the cuticle resist unnecessary swelling.

Most shampoos sold at drugstores and beauty supplies are pH balanced. It is standard practice for manufacturers to add citric acid or sodium citrate to adjust the pH of the product. Beware of shampoos made with soap or saponified oils because soap has a naturally high pH (around 8) that is particularly damaging for coils and curls. If you would like to test the pH of your shampoo at home, I recommend Micro Essentials pHydrion Plastic pH Indicator Strips, which you can purchase at Amazon.com.

Special Considerations

For color-treated hair: To make your color last as long as possible, choose a sulfate-free shampoo formulated for color-treated hair and only wash your hair twice a week maximum unless you have an oily scalp or dandruff.

For frequently heat-styled hair: Heat depletes natural oils from deep within the hair shaft. You may be tempted to shampoo your hair less because you want to make your straight hair last, but the only way to truly replenish moisture is to fully re-wet your hair at least every 7 days. Always cleanse thoroughly because residual dirt will burn (and smell bad) next time your hair is exposed to direct heat.

For relaxed hair: The majority of wear and tear that comes from washing relaxed hair happens when it swells with water. It is best to add a pre-shampoo oil treatment to your routine to minimize swelling damage. That way you can wash more often and enjoy more days of moisturized hair. Try the Pre-Shampoo Oil Treatment Tutorial in Chapter 7.

Shampoo Do's and Don'ts

Do start by rinsing your hair with warm water for about 3 minutes. The extra rinsing time will loosen up product residue so you can use less shampoo.

Don't comb your hair while you shampoo. Stretching and pulling creates unnecessary stress on your strands. Save detangling for when the conditioner is in.

Don't pile hair on top of your head because that will cause tangles. Apply the shampoo by smoothing it in a downward motion.

Don't underestimate the power of a high-quality shampoo; it can make all the difference.

Do shampoo your hair at least once a week. The health of your scalp determines how fast your hair grows. A healthy scalp is clean, flake-free and not itchy.

Recommended Shampoos Under $20

All of the shampoos recommended below are sulfate-free and safe for color-treated hair.

BEST BUY

L'Oreal EverCreme Intense Nourishing Shampoo

Available at drugstores, $7 for 8.5 oz.

You can't beat the price of this shampoo for the quality. A very small amount of product creates a rich, easy to spread lather. Look for the word "Intense" on the label to make sure you are getting the product with the most cationic conditioners.

Giovanni Colorflage Daily Color Defense Shampoo

Available at drugstores and online retailers, $9 for 8.5 oz.

This shampoo combines sulfate-free detergents, cationic conditioners, and "copolymers" which all help hair dye last longer.

Free Your Mane Sulfate Free Hydrating Shampoo

Available at FreeYourMane.com, $16 for 10.14 oz.

The Free Your Mane line of products was designed with coils and curls in mind. This shampoo lathers quickly and contains a high level of conditioners.

Carol's Daughter Chocolat Smoothing Shampoo

Available at Sephora and CarolsDaughter.com, $18 for 8.5 oz.

The Chocolat Smoothing Shampoo is the newest and best shampoo in the Carol's Daughter line.

CURLS Creamy Curl Cleanser

Available at Target and Sally Beauty $11 for 8 oz.

This cleansing cream is a great choice for those who prefer to wash daily because it contains very mild cleansers. It is definitely worth a try if co-washing does not agree with your scalp.

Joico Smooth Cure Sulfate-Free Shampoo

Available at beauty supply stores and online, $12 for 10.1 oz.

Smooth Cure is Joico's newest line of products for frizz-prone, curly hair. This shampoo includes all the important key ingredients along with hydrolyzed keratin to protect your hair from friction as you rub it with shampoo.

Find the Best Conditioners

Between washes your hair gets drier each day, the strands start to wrap around each other, and the volume starts to go to "the bad place". Your basic conditioner has one very important job to do and that is to make your hair easy to detangle. That is because coils and curls experience the least damage from combing when they are wet and saturated with conditioner. If you don't detangle your hair at least once a week, you may experience matting and tangles at your roots, which will be difficult to remove. Plus, once your hair has been thoroughly combed out, it will be easier to achieve your final style.

Conditioners that effectively detangle coils and curls contain:
• Emollients, which are conditioning ingredients that form a protective film on the hair and help your strands slide past each other as you detangle

• Cationic ingredients to condition your hair's cuticle

Emollients that offer good slip:

Dimethicone

Cyclopentasiloxane

Caprylic/Capric Triglyceride

Mineral Oil

Jojoba Oil

Cetyl Esters

Cetyl Alcohol*

Cetearyl Alcohol*

Stearyl Alcohol*

Cationic conditioners:

Amodimethicone

Behentrimonium Chloride

Behentrimonium Methosulfate

Cetrimonium Bromide

Cetrimonium Chloride

Cetrimonium Methosulfate

Guar Hydroxypropyltrimonium Chloride

Polyquaternium-7

Polyquaternium-37

Stearamidopropyl Dimethylamine

These are not the drying kinds of alcohol. They are called "fatty alcohols" and they'll help keep your hair soft and moisturized.

Special Considerations

For natural coils: African American coils are the most difficult to comb because of the way the hair naturally twists and turns. You can avoid breakage while detangling by choosing a conditioner that contains at least two emollients in the top 5.

For relaxed hair: Relaxed hair is easy to detangle until the new coils and curls grow in. Choose your staple conditioner by how well it performs when you have an inch or more of natural roots.

For frequently heat-styled hair: Heat protection starts with your conditioner. Look for basic conditioners that contain amodimethicone because it offers excellent heat protection. If you heat style your hair every week, it will be best to use a deep conditioner instead of a basic conditioner each wash. We will cover deep treatments in the next section.

Conditioning Do's and Don'ts

Do saturate your hair with conditioner from root to tip.

Don't ignore the inner layers of your hair. Distribute the conditioner as evenly as you would a relaxer.

Do comb the conditioner through before you rinse it out. Your scalp naturally sheds a small amount of hair each day and combing the conditioner through will help you remove any loose strands that have gotten "caught up".

Don't leave the conditioner on for longer than the maximum time in the instructions. The ingredients in rinse out conditioners are not meant to be left in contact with your skin for long periods.

Do comb out your hair by starting at the ends and working your way up to the roots. If you start from the roots, you will cause your ends to wrap around each other, which can lead to more tangles.

Is your conditioner a keeper?

If you can answer 'yes' to these questions after using a conditioner, go ahead and buy the largest bottle you can find. Conditioner is the product you will go through the fastest.

Did the comb glide through your hair as you detangled?
You have not found your conditioner match until you can comb through all of your hair within 5 minutes.

Was the conditioner easy to apply?
You have to condition every inch of every hair to get the best results. Choose a product that comes out of the bottle easily because that is a good indication that it will be easy to spread and distribute.

Recommended Conditioners Under $20

BEST BUY

Tresemme Naturals Nourishing Moisture Conditioner

Available at drugstores, $6 for 25 oz.

This conditioner has good slip to help you detangle in the shower, it spreads easily, and it contains a special "copolymer" that will help your hair retain moisture. It's a great place to start if you're on a tight budget.

John Frieda Full Repair Full Body Conditioner

Available at drugstores, $7 for 8.45 oz.

This product smoothes and detangles the hair without being too heavy. That is a difficult combination to find in a drugstore conditioner. Some stores also sell a 20 oz. size that comes with a pump, which is helpful when you have a lot of hair to work through.

Dove Nourishing Oil Care Daily Treatment Conditioner

Available at drugstores, $5 for 12 oz.

Dove's Nourishing Oil Care conditioner combines silicone oil (dimethicone), coconut oil, and mineral oil to deliver maximum slip.

Free Your Mane Daily Detangling Conditioner

Available at FreeYourMane.com, $16 for 10.14 oz.

This conditioner spreads easily and has enough slip to get through stubborn tangles. It also contains extra ingredients that give lasting shine and smoothness to the hair.

Joico Smooth Cure Conditioner

Available at beauty supply stores and online, $14 for 10.1 oz.

Joico Smooth Cure conditioner and the matching shampoo make a worthwhile combo for hair that gets heat-styled often. The conditioner has a combination of emollients, cationics, and hydrolyzed keratin, so it also qualifies as a deep treatment.

Pantene Pro-V Restore Beautiful Lengths Shine Enhance Conditioner

Available at drugstores, $6 for 8.5 oz.

This conditioner will leave your hair noticeably shinier, which can help you blend your new growth if your hair is chemically-treated. It may not have enough slip to detangle natural coils.

Find the Best Deep Treatments

Coils and curls need constant TLC because each styling session leaves your hair weaker than the day before. Regular use of a deep treatment will patch and smooth your strands so you can enjoy your length instead of always having to cut it off.

The most effective deep conditioning treatments contain:
• Hydrolyzed protein to strengthen your hair against breakage
• Cationic conditioners to make your hair easier to comb
• Emollients to smooth and soften the cuticle

Hydrolyzed Protein

Look at a strand of your hair. Eighty percent of what you are looking at is keratin protein. Your body uses the protein you eat to create keratin protein for your hair and skin. You really are feeding your hair and skin whenever you eat eggs, meat, and certain vegetables. Adding more protein to your diet can strengthen the hair that is currently being "built". However, once a hair emerges from its follicle, your health and what you eat does not affect its appearance anymore. Your hair is at your mercy and daily combing and styling chip away tiny pieces of keratin from each strand. It is up to you to replace those lost pieces with protein and other moisturizing ingredients from hair products; otherwise, your hair may break just as fast as it grows. If you have been stuck at shoulder length, one of the first things you can do is make sure your deep treatment contains hydrolyzed protein. In cosmetic labs, scientists "hydrolyze" proteins from plants and animals to make them substantive to your hair. The term "hydrolyzed" means the protein are small enough to fit in the spaces between your hair's cuticle layers. Usually, you get the most benefit from an ingredient if it is in the top 5, but hydrolyzed protein is a little bit different. Cosmetic scientists often add "helper" ingredients to make lower amounts of protein more effective, so do not rule out a product just because hydrolyzed protein is not at the beginning of the list.

Examples of hydrolyzed protein:

Hydrolyzed Keratin (from wool)

Hydrolyzed Oat Protein

Hydrolyzed Silk Protein

Hydrolyzed Soy Protein

Hydrolyzed Vegetable Protein

Hydrolyzed Wheat Protein

Cationic Conditioners

Deep treatments need to perform double duty. Protein will strengthen your hair, but it could still snap from basic combing. Deep conditioners that contain cationics will condition the cuticle and make your hair easier to comb.

Cationic conditioners often found in deep treatments:

Amodimethicone

Behentrimonium Chloride

Behentrimonium Methosulfate

Cetrimonium Bromide

Cetrimonium Chloride

Cetrimonium Methosulfate

Guar Hydroxypropyltrimonium Chloride

Polyquaternium-7

Polyquaternium-37

Stearamidopropyl Dimethylamine

Emollients

Without emollients, your conditioner will leave your hair moisturized and easier to comb, but probably not as smooth as you would like. The emollients listed below will leave your hair looking smooth and feeling soft. They will also help your strands retain moisture as you style your hair.

Emollients to look for in deep treatments:

Dimethicone

Glyceryl Stearate

Jojoba Oil

Mineral Oil

Petrolatum

Phenyl Trimethicone

Shea Butter

Special Considerations

For color-treated hair: Permanent color treatments lift the hair's cuticle and make it more porous. Always deep condition your hair the last time you shampoo before your color appointment and the first time you shampoo after your appointment.

For frequently heat-styled hair: Your hair will be easiest to comb and style if you shampoo and deep condition every time you plan to heat-style. Make sure your deep treatment also has good slip so you won't need a separate product to detangle your hair.

For relaxed hair: Relaxed hair is easily weighed down so choose treatments that contain lightweight synthetic oils like dimethicone or phenyl trimethicone. Definitely deep condition before and after each touch-up.

3 Key Tips for Deep Conditioning

1 Always shampoo your hair before applying a deep treatment. If you only co-wash or rinse before you apply the product, your hair won't be able to absorb as much hydrolyzed protein.

2 Follow the instructions on your product. The best deep treatments contain a careful blend of ingredients that will give you maximum benefits in 30 minutes or less. Do not put off deep conditioning because you don't have time to sit under the dryer. That is usually unnecessary and you will end up deep conditioning your hair less often.

3 Only condition the hair you want to keep! Choose a deep conditioner that you can afford to use generously. It won't matter if your product is filled with great ingredients if you don't apply it to every inch of your hair.

Have you found a deep conditioner match?

If you can answer 'yes' to all of these questions, you've found a staple.

Was the product easy to apply?

There is no reason that a deep treatment has to be very thick. It is easier to control the amount you use if the product spreads easily.

Could you at least finger comb your hair after rinsing the treatment out?

The most efficient products do not require you to follow-up with a separate conditioner. If you can do your full detangling routine, you really have a winner.

Do you see significantly less broken hair than usual?

After your shower, detangle your most breakage prone (shortest) section with your fingers. If you have found the right product for your hair, breakage should drastically decrease after one use and continue to improve. You will have to keep using the product regularly (or one very similar) to keep breakage at bay.

Recommended Deep Treatments Under $30

Deep conditioners are often more expensive than other products, but that does not mean you have to spend a lot. Check the ingredients lists of products made for "dry/damaged hair" and look for sales and coupons to get the best bargains.

BEST BUY

Nuance Salma Hayek Blackcurrant Intense Hydration Hair Mask

Available at CVS Drugstores, $10 for 8 oz.

This mask combines hydrolyzed protein, cationic conditioners, and a touch of shea butter. It spreads easily, so a little goes a long way. Maximum results require 20 minutes (without heat).

Age Beautiful Strengthening Treatment

Available at Sally Beauty, $10 for 5.1 oz.

This treatment won the Good Housekeeping Research Institute's highest award for deep conditioners in 2011. It is a steal for color-treated and relaxed hair because it contains a special copolymer that helps repair cuticle damage from chemical treatments. Even if you don't make it your staple, it's a good product to keep around for immediately after touch-ups.

ApHogee Two-Step Protein Treatment (Step 1), $9 for 4 oz. and **ApHogee Balancing Moisturizer** (Step 2), $6 for 8 oz. Available at Sally Beauty

ApHogee Two-Step Protein Treatment has been around for years. This is an effective and affordable treatment but it has an unpleasant smell and the protein step can get messy. If you are on a very tight budget, it is a good place to start. This product requires 5-10 minutes under a hooded dryer. Make sure to follow the instructions exactly as written or you could end up with unnecessary breakage.

Joico K-PAK RevitaLuxe Bio-Advanced Restorative Treatment

Available at drugstores and beauty supply stores, $23 for 5.1 oz. The "bio-advanced" part of this treatment refers to peptides (similar to proteins) that are used to help decrease inflammation on the scalp and promote hair growth. There is good scientific evidence for the effect of peptides on the skin, so this product is worth a try if you have had a history of scalp problems.

Carol's Daughter Monoi Repairing Hair Mask

Available at Sephora and CarolsDaughter.com, $29 for 7 oz. Carol's Daughter Monoi Repairing Hair Mask has all the requisite ingredients for a good deep conditioning treatment plus good slip. Maximum benefits require 10 to 15 minutes of heat.

Leave-In Products

How Thick Are Your Strands?

It takes just the right blend of moisturizing ingredients and emollients to tame coils and curls. The emollients are the tricky part. Too heavy and they will weigh your hair down, too light and you will end up with frizz. To find the right leave-ins for your hair, it is important that you understand your "strand thickness", which can be categorized as "fine to medium" or "medium to thick". When you see those words on a product label, they are not referring to how much hair you have; they are describing the thickness of each individual strand on your head. The words "coarse" and "thick" are used interchangeably, but they both refer to the size of individual strands of hair.

Your ethnic background does not determine your "strand thickness". Two women may have similar looking coils, but one woman's strands might be twice the size of the others. The only way to know exactly where your hair falls would be to visit a trichologist or dermatologist who has a special microscope that measures strand size. Fine hairs are around 60 micrometers in diameter; thick hairs are around 100 micrometers. However, you do not need to be that exact. The telltale sign of fine hair is thick-looking roots with a thin-looking ponytail. If you have fine hair, you are likely to have a lot of strands. Those strands look nice and dense near the roots, but as the hair grows longer, the relative thinness of the strands becomes more noticeable. The strand thickness slightly varies on different parts of your head, so it can still be difficult to decide how to categorize your hair. Don't worry about getting too specific, you just need a general idea, so you can find products that make your hair look and feel the way you want.

Choose your leave-in conditioners and stylers based on the emollients that you see in the top 5. If you think your strands are fine to medium, choose products that contain lightweight emollients. If you think your strands are on the thicker side, look for products that contain heavier emollients. Whether you are using a leave-in conditioner or styler, you need to be able to distribute the product evenly, from root to tip, without worrying that it will leave your hair looking greasy.

Lighter Emollients For Fine to Medium Thickness:	Heavier Emollients For Medium to Coarse Thickness:
Argan Oil	Avocado Oil
C12-15 Alkyl Benzoate	Castor Oil
Dimethicone*	Cetyl Esters
Grape Seed Oil	Cocoa Butter
Mango Butter	Coconut Oil
Phenyl Trimethicone*	Jojoba Esters
Soybean Oil	Jojoba Oil
Sunflower Oil	Olive Oil
Sweet Almond Oil	Mineral Oil
	Shea Butter

*Dimethicone and phenyl trimethicone leave the hair shinier than other ingredients so keep an eye out for those if you want glossy coils and curls.

It will take some trial and error to find leave-ins that you love. Many products contain a combination of emollients and more sophisticated ingredients like polymers and cationic conditioners. This is a good time to read the rest of the label, not just the ingredients list. The descriptions on leave-in products usually mention "fine" or "thick/coarse" hair

Pure Oils and Butters

Benefits and Recipe Ideas

I recommend that you only begin incorporating oils and butters into your routine after you have found your favorite commercial products. Pure oils and butters are better to use before or after you wash your hair because unlike cationic conditioners which are substantive (strongly attracted to your hair), most oils will go down the drain when you rinse. The plant-based emollients listed below have unique properties that make them beneficial for your hair and skin.

Coconut Oil

Coconut is the best pure oil to apply to your hair because it contains "lauric acid", a fatty acid that is naturally attracted to keratin protein. To do an effective oil treatment, you must apply the oil before you shampoo. The lauric acid allows a small amount of coconut oil to absorb into your strands once you wet your hair. The oil that remains on your hair after you shampoo will help you detangle with your conditioner. If your hair is relaxed or color-treated, the coconut oil will also prevent your strands from swelling excessively when they get wet, which is a significant cause of damage for chemically-treated hair.

Jojoba Oil

The composition of jojoba oil makes it very similar to the sebum produced by our hair follicles. Jojoba oil is technically a liquid wax, which lets you know it is a little bit heavier than other "oils". You can use jojoba oil to massage your scalp before you shampoo. That may be beneficial because your hair follicles can be clogged just like the pores on your face. Jojoba oil will penetrate into your hair follicles and loosen up clogs to leave you with a healthier scalp. If you don't usually have scalp problems, pre-shampoo massages are probably unnecessary. You can also add a little bit of jojoba oil to your conditioner if it doesn't have enough slip.

Shea Butter

Shea butter is a powerful emollient because it contains allantoin, a unique component that helps water stay trapped inside the hair and skin for longer periods. Shea butter is considered a heavy emollient, so it is best used in stylers for medium-thick strands. You can also use it sparingly as a pomade (a small dab at a time) to smooth fly aways on any hair type.

Recipe Ideas

For a pre-shampoo scalp massage:

1 tablespoon jojoba oil

3 drops of tea tree oil (or the essential oil of your choice)

For a pre-shampoo oil treatment:

4 tablespoons of coconut oil (warm it in the microwave for about 10 seconds to make it easier to spread)

To add more slip to your conditioner:

1 part jojoba oil

3 parts rinse-out conditioner

For a styler or pomade:

2 parts shea butter

1 part coconut oil

3 Tips for Using Pure Oils and Butters

1 Buy small amounts of oils and butters until you find your favorites. A little goes a long way.

2 Store your oils and butters in a cabinet outside of the bathroom. The heat and steam from your shower will make your oil go bad faster. Expired oils are sticky and they give off a sour smell.

3 For a DIY alternative to body lotion, apply coconut oil or whipped shea butter while your skin is still damp from the shower.

Product Safety

5 Ways to Protect Your Health

Product safety is something I take very seriously. Over recent years, we have heard many warnings about parabens, phthalates, BPA…the list goes on and on. Ignorance is really bliss because once you start learning about the risks of personal care products it starts to seem like nothing is safe. I say "personal care" because this issue is not limited to hair products. The same chemicals are used in hair and skin products; some of them are even allowed in food.

A few personal care chemicals that are currently in question:

Dioxane

Nitrosamines

Parabens

Phthalates

You will not see the first two chemicals on any ingredients list because they are byproducts of the manufacturing process and therefore are not required to be included in the product's ingredients list. Think of it this way, if you often leave a bit of egg shell in the batter when you make cookies, that doesn't mean you'll include "egg shells" when someone asks for the recipe. Product manufacturing is not a perfect process either and FDA regulations do not require companies to "tell all".

There are five important things you can do to limit your exposure to personal care chemicals:

1 Limit the number of products you use on a daily basis. Can you get it down to less than 10? That would include everything from toothpaste to perfume. The fewer products you use, the better.

2 Pay the most attention to the products that you leave on your skin. Some chemicals are not harmful when they are rinsed off, but they cause problems when they are left on. This is the most important reason not to leave conditioner on your hair and scalp for longer than the maximum time in the instructions.

3 Always wash your hands with soap and water after applying personal care products. A chemical's ability to cause you harm depends on which areas of your body it comes into contact with and for how long. If you apply your products and then proceed to rub your eyes, touch your mouth, cook dinner, etc. You are increasing your risk of exposure.

4 Minimize the number of store brought products you use on children. Just like with certain foods, pregnant women and children need to be most careful. With that said, it is important to use products that deliver results so that your children can grow up understanding how to work with their coils and curls. CURLS, Free Your Mane, Kinky-Curly and Mixed Chicks make my favorite hair products for kids. You can replace other products like lotion and lip balm with homemade mixes.

5 If you have a bad reaction to a product (a rash for example), report the problem through the FDA website. You may be able to prevent other people from having a bad (or worse) experience if you speak up.

More Product Safety Resources:
FDA For Consumers: www.fda.gov/ForConsumers

Environmental Working Group's Skin Deep Cosmetics Database: www.ewg.org/skindeep

In my opinion, it is best to start by finding the products that will help you care and style for your hair with the least amount of time and frustration. You can look for alternatives after you know what good results look like.

Product Cheat Sheets

Check for these products and ingredients next time to you head to the store

Recommended Hair Products

Drugstore Best Buys

- Shampoo - L'Oreal EverCreme Intense Nourishing Shampoo
- Conditioner - Tresemme Naturals Nourishing Moisture Conditioner
- Deep Treatment - Nuance Salma Hayek Blackcurrant Intense Hydration Hair Mask

Recommended Shampoos

- Giovanni Colorflage Daily Color Defense Shampoo
- Free Your Mane Sulfate Free Hydrating Shampoo
- Carol's Daughter Chocolat Smoothing Shampoo
- CURLS Creamy Curl Cleanser
- Joico Smooth Cure Sulfate-Free Shampoo

Recommended Conditioners

- Dove Damage Therapy Nourishing Oil Care Daily Treatment Conditioner
- John Frieda Full Repair Full Body Conditioner
- Free Your Mane Daily Detangling Conditioner
- Joico Smooth Cure Conditioner

Recommended Deep Treatments

- Age Beautiful Strengthening Treatment
- ApHogee Two-Step Protein Treatment (Step 1) and ApHogee Balancing Moisturizer (Step 2)
- Joico K-PAK RevitaLuxe Bio-Advanced Restorative Treatment
- Carol's Daughter Monoi Repairing Hair Mask

Key Ingredients by Product

Shampoos

Amodimethicone

Citric Acid

Coco-Glucoside

Decyl Glucoside

Disodium Cocoamphodipropionate

Disodium Laureth Sulfosuccinate

Disodium Lauroamphodiacetate

Guar Hydroxypropyltrimonium Chloride

Polyquaternium-7

Polyquaternium-10

Polyquaternium-11

Polyquaternium-44

Polyquaternium-47

Sodium Citrate

Sodium Cocoyl Isethionate

Sodium Methyl Cocoyl Taurate

Conditioners and Deep Treatments

Amodimethicone

Behentrimonium Chloride

Behentrimonium Methosulfate

Caprylic/Capric Triglyceride

Cetearyl Alcohol

Cetrimonium Bromide

Cetrimonium Chloride

Cetrimonium Methosulfate

Cetyl Alcohol

Cetyl Esters

Cyclopentasiloxane

Dimethicone

Guar Hydroxypropyltrimonium Chloride

Hydrolyzed Keratin

Hydrolyzed Oat Protein

Hydrolyzed Silk Protein

Hydrolyzed Soy Protein

Hydrolyzed Vegetable Protein

Hydrolyzed Wheat Protein

Jojoba Oil

Mineral Oil

Petrolatum

Phenyl Trimethicone

Polyquaternium-7

Polyquaternium-10

Polyquaternium-11

Polyquaternium-32

Polyquaternium-37

Shea Butter

Stearamidopropyl Dimethylamine

Stearyl Alcohol

It's impossible to list all the ingredients that are beneficial for your hair. You will see many other ingredients listed as you read labels. When you find a product you love, stick with it. The results come from a specific recipe that may be hard to imitate.

④

The Staple Product Formula

Even when you shop smart, some of the best products still seem expensive. I developed this simple formula to help you decide if you can afford to incorporate a pricey product into your routine

Put that product sample to work!

Have fun trying new products by picking up sample sizes. If you like the results you get, follow these steps to figure out how much it would cost you to use the product every month.

Step 1: Purchase a sample of the product. Samples are usually 1 to 2 ounces.

Step 2: See how many uses you get out of the sample. Depending on your hair length and thickness, you will probably get 1-3 uses out of a 2 oz. bottle.

Step 3: Divide the size of the sample by the number of uses you got out of it. If a 2 oz. sample resulted in two uses, you used 1 oz. each time.

Step 4: If you like the results you get from the sample check the price of the largest bottle you can afford. Usually, the larger the size you buy, the lower the price per ounce.

Use this formula to see if you can afford to make
the product one of your staples:

(Cost of largest bottle you can afford) × (# of ounces used each time)
$$\frac{\times \text{(# of times per week you plan to use the product)}}{\text{Size of largest bottle you can afford, in ounces}}$$

Example using a new deep treatment I am considering:

$$\frac{(\$35 \times 1 \times 1)}{16} = \$2.20 \text{ per week} = \$9 \text{ per month}$$

Since the product spreads well, I only need to use
one ounce each time and it is a deep treatment so
I won't use it as quickly as I would a styling
product. For $9 a month, it looks like I can try it
without breaking the bank. If I had just looked at
the price, I might have ruled it out. You can use
this formula to help you evaluate samples as you
try them. Once you know what ingredients to
look for, you can find the combination of
products that make your hair look and feel great
without over-spending.

Hair Care How To's

Most of us just want to wear our hair down. It sounds so simple, but sometimes it seems impossible to do more than a few days a month! Once you have the right hair products, you are more than half way there, but your styling routine is important too. Take advantage of all the new tools and techniques that have emerged over recent years so you can enjoy more time whipping your hair.

Updates to Old School Hair Care

Some old school methods of hair care are damaging and need to be left in the past; others have stood the test of time.

Old School Method: Hot Combs

Hot combs are metal combs that heat on a home stovetop or in a professional ceramic stove. They used to be the go-to tool to straighten African American hair. Electric hot combs are also available.

Why Hot Combs worked

Hot combs were used for decades before relaxers were invented. Ceramic stoves can heat the hot comb up to 400-500 °F, which is more than enough heat to transform tight natural coils to stick straight hair with one or two strokes.

Why Hot Combs are old school

Pressing combs can cause severe heat damage. Healthy coils and curls usually have a similar texture throughout but just a few styling sessions with a hot comb can leave the hair permanently and unevenly straighter. Some call that "heat-training" the hair. Heat damage is irreversible, which means once your natural texture is gone you will not be able to get it back. Sadly, hair products cannot "repair" or "define" heat-damaged coils and curls (so don't waste your money!).

Heat damage takes away some of your hair's versatility. When you end up with multiple textures, you have to choose between straight styles or wet-sets. Both options take much more time than a curly wash 'n go or quick twist-out. Hot combs should never be used on relaxed hair because the high heat can cause immediate breakage.

The Modern Choice: Ceramic flat irons

To get sleek, straight hair without ruining your natural texture, it is best to use a ceramic flat iron. Flat irons press your hair between two smooth plates that heat more evenly and quickly than hot combs. Most natural hair can be straightened with a setting between 350 °F and 400 °F. Relaxed hair responds to heat as low as 300 °F. The trick with a flat iron is to get as close to your roots as you would with a pressing comb. Take sections about 1" wide and pull the hair taut before you iron it (just as you would if you were ironing a shirt).

Old School Method: Petrolatum and mineral oil based products

This includes all styling products that contain petrolatum, mineral oil or any type of wax in the top 5 ingredients. Examples include Blue Magic, Luster's Pink Oil Moisturizer, Organic Root Stimulator Olive Oil Nourishing Sheen Spray, and Clairol Vitapointe. Back in the day, petrolatum and mineral oil based products laid down fly aways and made our hair shine better than anything else could.

Why petrolatum and mineral oil based products worked

Petrolatum, mineral oil, and wax are heavy emollients. Emollients are ingredients that leave a smooth, soft coating on the hair. Heavy emollients literally weigh the hair down with a thick coating that smoothes the cuticle.

Why petrolatum and mineral oil-based products are old school

The heavy, greasy look that comes from petrolatum and mineral oil is outdated. If you have relaxed hair or fine-medium natural hair, those old school products will quickly leave your strands looking thin and stiff. To get soft, fluffy hair, most women want products light enough to smooth the cuticle without leaving an oily residue. If you have thicker strands, you might like the effect petrolatum and mineral oil based products have on your hair. If so, you should definitely continue using them.

The Modern Alternative: Silicone oils

Decades of scientific research have made it possible to get the benefits of petrolatum and mineral oil based products without the greasiness. In 1998, cosmetic manufacturers began replacing the heavy emollients in hair products with the lighter types of emollients they were using in skin products. The newer lightweight ·
emollients are called "silicone oils". Silicones are synthetic (man-made) oils. Examples include dimethicone, dimethiconol,

cyclopentasiloxane, and phenyl trimethicone. Silicone oils are also used in lotions, face creams, and skin medications. These days, hair products from almost every brand contain silicones including Motions, Carol's Daughter, Miss Jessie's, Pantene, and many more. To learn more about silicones, please read the article, "Synthetic Oils to Combat Dry Hair" at HairLiberty.org.

Old School Method: Protective Styling

Mum Oprah (as I like to call her) explained this old school method to Chris Rock on her talk show in 2009. She said, "I have worn weaves, I have worn wigs, I have done all of it, because in order to keep your hair, you can't put heat on your hair every day! You have to give your hair a break." Protective styles like braids, twists, wigs, and weaves are often used to give ethnic hair an extended break from daily combing and heat styling.

Why Protective Styling works

Coils and curls are more likely to be damaged by simple combing and styling than any other hair type. Fine to medium strands also break more easily than thicker strands. If your hair starts to break constantly once it reaches shoulder length that means it is being damaged at the ends faster than it grows at the roots. Protective styles allow you to slow down the damage cycle by not combing your hair for a few weeks at a time.

Why Protective Styling is optional

This old school method still makes sense, but it is not a requirement for growing long coils and curls. If a protective style is put in too tight and/or left in for too long, it can do more harm than good. The hair can become matted and brittle from not being thoroughly washed and when it's time for the style to come out, the length retained during the rest period can be ripped away by one rough combing session. Current scientific research shows that tight styles that are left in for long periods cause stress on the scalp that can lead to permanent hair loss.

The Modern Option: Protective products

You can slow down the damage cycle by using products that not only condition, but also protect your hair from heat and combing. If you choose your products using the recommendations in this book, you will be free to rock whatever style you want, whenever you want. Ingredients like cationic conditioners, silicones, and hydrolyzed protein will patch and protect your hair with every use so you don't have to limit your style choices. It will always be important to comb your hair as little as possible, but the days when you had to "put your hair away" in order to grow it long are over!

Celebrate the Versatility of your

Coils & Curls

These sample routines will help you get on the fast
track to healthy hair

No More Breakage Natural Hair Routine

COMB. The 4-letter curse word when it comes to natural coils and curls. The curlier your strands, the more likely you are to see short broken pieces when you comb (or brush) your hair, especially when it is dry. However, that breakage is preventable. The ingredients that you learned about in Chapter 2 are all designed to make your hair easier to comb and they need to be applied evenly and often. You will know that you have found the right combination of products when you can detangle your hair in the shower within 5 minutes. No matter how thick, kinky, or dry your hair usually seems, with the right products, detangling should be very, very easy. If it's not, you'll experience unnecessary breakage as you wash and style your hair.

I have included a "Wash N Wear" regimen for natural hair because I want to help you develop a routine that delivers the most moisture and the least combing. A strand of hair can hold a maximum amount of 14% water. When your natural coils and curls are looking their best, the moisture level is likely to be close to its optimum level. But, each day between washes your strands get drier and they may start to become brittle. You can re-moisturize with products, but once your hair drops below 10% moisture, it is like a stiff, dried out sponge.

The best way to fully re-moisturize and restore your hair's elasticity is to saturate it with water in the shower. Depending on your climate, you may need to do that every few hours or every few days. Try keeping track of how easy it is to style your hair and whether or not you can do so without breakage. If you start to get stubborn tangles or breakage from lightly touching your hair, it's time to re-moisturize in the shower by shampooing or co-washing. By following the Wash N Wear routine and product recommendations in this book, you can wash your hair multiple times each week and watch it thrive.

If your coils and curls are losing their natural shape at the ends, you will need to "transition" into a Wash N Wear routine. Natural hair is stronger than relaxed hair, but it is still highly prone to damage. Even when you have given up chemical treatments, heat styling can cause loss of curl if it is done at too high of a temperature. Although there are some very effective products on the market today, none can restore your strands to their original texture after they have become wavy or straight. You can camouflage those areas with wet sets and/or updos until you are ready to have them trimmed away.

My advice is to plan for two go-to styles that you can stick with for a few months at a time. Choose styles that are easy for you to do at your current length and then re-assess in 2-3 months when your hair is slightly longer. Once you have a consistent curl pattern throughout, it will be easier to Wash N Wear without hiding or manipulating the ends. The sooner you can limit all of your combing to the shower, the better your coils and curls will look in their natural state.

Weekly Routine for Natural Coils & Curls

WASH DAY

- Start each wash by rinsing your hair for 2-3 minutes. The long rinse will loosen up product residue so you can use less shampoo.

- Comb the conditioner through your hair before rinsing it out. Coils and curls experience the least damage when they are covered in conditioner.

- Be sure to "lock" in your curl pattern with a leave-in conditioner and/or a curl styler while you can still see it (i.e. when your hair is still very wet).

Weekly Routine for Natural Coils & Curls

DAILY

- When your hair is at its optimal moisture level, it can handle light touching and pulling without breaking. If you start to see little broken hairs between washes, that is a sign that you need to re-moisturize your hair ASAP. You can choose to shampoo and condition, just condition (co-wash), or apply more of your leave-in products. You will have to decide what strategy leads to the least breakage for you.

- It is important to shampoo your hair whenever you sweat. The sweat that comes from your pores contains bacteria that can lead to scalp irritation and slower hair growth. Don't be afraid to shampoo and condition your hair as often as necessary. When you are using the right products and techniques, washing is helpful, not harmful, for your coils and curls.

Weekly Routine for Natural Coils & Curls

1 TO 4 TIMES EACH MONTH

- Co-washing does not cleanse your scalp enough to keep it healthy. Shampoo your hair at least twice a month or whenever it's starting to look dull.

- Deep Condition your hair as often as possible. Saturate every inch of hair with your deep treatment and leave it in for the full recommended time.

Weekly Routine for Natural Coils & Curls

5 Tips for a Successful "Wash N Wear"

1 Don't comb or brush your hair after you rinse out the conditioner or your natural coils and curls will frizz out and seem to disappear.

2 Practice applying your products to your wet hair in the shower. To get the best results, you need to lock in your curl pattern before the "puff" sets in. Think seconds, not minutes! After you have distributed the product evenly from roots to ends, gently towel blot any areas that are dripping.

3 If your usual styling product is actually a rinse out conditioner, it would be best to switch to a product that's meant to be left in. Look for a leave-in conditioner that has "cetearyl alcohol" and another emollient in the top 5.

4 Visit the DIY section at HairLiberty.org to learn how to elongate and define your natural hair with a blow dryer and minimal heat.

5 Careful product application is the key to a successful "Wash N Wear". If you have tight coils, smooth the product through your very wet hair row-by-row, starting at the roots.

Weekly Routine for Natural Coils & Curls

Products & Tools Required

Shampoo

Conditioner

Deep Treatment

Curl Styler and/or Leave-In Conditioner

Wide Tooth Comb

Blow Dryer & Diffuser

Leave-In Products to Try

For Fine-Medium Strands

- AG Hair Fast Food Leave On Conditioner
- As I Am Smoothing Gel
- Curls Cashmere Curl Jelly
- Hair Rules Curly Whip

For Medium-Thick Strands

- Beautiful Textures Curl Control Defining Pudding
- Curls Whipped Cream
- Hair Rules Kinky Curling Cream
- Miss Jessie's Stretch Silkening Crème

Texture Taming Relaxed Hair Regimen

Chemical relaxers were created to make coils and curls easier to comb and style. If you prefer to wear your hair straight most of the time, a properly applied relaxer will allow you to use less heat on your hair each week, which will keep it healthier. The newest professional relaxer systems now include pre-treatments that contain cationic conditioners to help the hair maintain more of its original strength than previous formulas. The challenge these days lies in the way that relaxers are applied. A section of hair should be relaxed once and only once. Problems often arise after multiple touch-ups have been done and the previously relaxed hair has become weaker and drier.

First, it is critically important to have the relaxer applied by an educated professional that understands your goals for healthy hair. It is best not to relax your hair until it's "bone straight", especially if you plan to heat-style it anyway. Ask your stylist to leave some of your hair's natural texture intact. After that, it is up to you to keep your strands moisturized and protected so you can wait until you have 1 to 2 inches of new growth before you make a touch-up appointment. That may take anywhere from

10 to 16 weeks. Giving your stylist "extra room to work" will minimize overlapping of the chemical and scalp irritation. Burns on your scalp, even those that seem minor, can cause damage to your follicles that will affect the way your coils and curls look as they grow in. Also, keep in mind that no-lye relaxers can be helpful if you have a sensitive scalp, but they are not gentler on your hair than lye relaxers.

Careful product selection will help you keep your relaxed hair looking healthy. Choose lightweight leave-in products that contain ceramides and/or amino acids because those ingredients will help you prevent damage from basic styling. Coils and curls are already more porous than other hair types, and relaxers are inherently damaging. Relaxed hair is particularly prone to excessive swelling whenever it is saturated with water. Hair that swells quickly to take in water and contracts quickly to let that water go eventually begins to fray at the ends like a worn out rubber band. When you have time to give your hair extra TLC, do an oil treatment before you shampoo. The oil will prevent your hair from excessive swelling so you can keep your length longer instead of having to cut it off.

Weekly Routine for Relaxed Hair

WASH DAY

- Start each wash by rinsing your hair for 2-3 minutes. The long rinse will loosen up product residue so you can use less shampoo.

- Comb the conditioner through your hair before rinsing it out. This will be best time to comb through any new growth you have.

- Apply a leave-in conditioner immediately after you towel blot your hair. Focus more product on the roots as they grow out.

- If you plan to heat-style your hair, apply a heat protection foam or serum immediately after your leave-in conditioner.

Weekly Routine for Relaxed Hair

DAILY

- Moisturize your hair by using more leave-in conditioner. Apply the product sparingly to avoid overloading your strands between washes.

MID-WEEK OR MORE OFTEN

- If you heat-styled your hair on wash day, you may be tempted to touch up your ends with a flat iron or curling iron. Don't do it! In order to keep your hair from becoming brittle, you should avoid using heat between washes.

- To bring the bounce back to your ends, moisturize and roll large sections of your hair with curlers before you shower. Don't forget to cover everything with a scarf before you put on your shower cap.

- Feel free to shampoo or co-wash if your hair starts to feel very dry.

Weekly Routine for Relaxed Hair

1 TO 4 TIMES PER MONTH

- Do an oil treatment before you shampoo. The majority of wear and tear that comes from washing relaxed hair happens when it swells with water. Pre-shampoo oil treatments minimize swelling damage so you can wash your hair more often.

- Deep condition your hair as often as possible. Always saturate every inch of hair with your deep treatment and leave it in for the full recommended time.

Weekly Routine for Relaxed Hair

4 Heat Styling Tips

1 Lessen the amount of heat you put on your hair by air drying after you apply your leave-in products (don't air dry without applying products first). It is best to skip the blow dryer whenever possible, especially if you find a lot of broken hair on your shoulders after using it.

2 Straighten your hair using a ceramic flat iron with a temperature control. Always use just enough heat that you only need to do 1 or 2 passes.

3 Practice heat-free styles like wet sets and updos so you can give your hair time to recover from your usual straightening process.

4 Wrap, pin curl, or braid your hair at night to keep it smooth and minimize breakage. The better you protect your hair at night, the less you will have to do each morning.

Weekly Routine for Relaxed Hair

Products & Tools Required

Shampoo

Conditioner

Deep Treatment

Leave-In Conditioner

Heat Protection Foam or Serum

Bobby Pins and/or Rollers

Wide Tooth Comb

Ceramic Flat Iron

Satin Scarf

Leave-In Products to Try

- Carol's Daughter Macadamia Heat Setting Foam
- CHI Silk Infusion Silk Reconstructing Complex
- Living Proof Restore Targeted Repair Cream
- Smooth 'N Shine Silk Style Foaming Wrap Lotion
- Softsheen Carson Optimum Care Salon Collection Heat Protection Polisher

Straight-to-Curly Grow Out Strategy

Growing out a permanent chemical treatment requires patience and planning. If you are growing out a relaxer (or some other permanent straightener), your new growth will be thicker and curlier than your ends, which means your roots will be more difficult to comb. As you let your natural coils and curls grow out, keep in mind that the hair you will be "keeping" the longest is at your roots, not at your ends. Take every precaution to condition and protect your new growth. The chemically-treated ends will be cut off sooner than later, but your "new" growth will be around for years.

I think you will want to focus your styling efforts on blending your different textures, so I have included a routine for weekly wet sets. Styles like roller sets and twists outs allow you to do the majority of the "work" on wash day which makes the rest of the week much easier. When you first start growing out your chemical treatment, stick with the same leave-in products you have already been using. As your new coils and curls grow out, you may want to switch to products that contain heavier emollients and more smoothing power. Your hair will be constantly changing, so plan to re-evaluate your leave-ins every few months. If you prefer to flat iron your hair during the grow out phase (be forewarned that you may compromise your natural curl pattern before you get a chance to see it), follow the Texture Taming Relaxed Hair Regimen and opt for heat-free styles whenever possible.

You may be nervous about having some bad hair days and that is completely understandable, especially if you have not worked with your natural texture in a while. It can't hurt to keep a wig or some clip-in hair pieces nearby "in case of emergency". Do whatever you need to do to feel pretty!

Weekly Routine for Growing Out a Relaxer

WASH DAY

- Shampoo and deep condition your hair every week to avoid knots and matting at your roots.

- Choose a deep treatment that you can use in the shower and use it as often as possible.

- Comb the conditioner through before rinsing it out. This is the best time to thoroughly detangle your hair with minimal damage.

- Apply a leave-in conditioner immediately after you towel blot your hair. The more new growth you have, the more important it will become to apply your products when your hair is still wet (not damp).

Weekly Routine for Growing Out a Relaxer

DAILY

- Moisturize once a day with more leave-in conditioner. Apply extra product at your roots to keep them smooth and "tame".

- Keep a shine serum or spray on hand to smooth fly aways. Extra shine will make the contrast in your textures less noticeable.

MID-WEEK OR MORE OFTEN

- Those with oily scalps or a frequent exercise schedule will need to shampoo mid-week. If you don't have the time to roller set, opt for a Twist-Out or Braid-Out.

- If you have medium-thick strands, try co-washing midweek instead of your full shampoo and deep condition routine. If you have finer hair, co-washing may leave your straight ends looking dull and thin.

- Whether you re-wash your hair or not, you can change up your look with an updo. Visit the DIY section at HairLiberty.org for style ideas.

Weekly Routine for Growing Out a Relaxer

3 Tips for Growing Out a Relaxer

1 Do your best to avoid high heat. Wet sets will prevent you from unevenly loosening your natural coils and curls with heat. If you decide to straighten your hair, the best way to prevent damage is to keep the flat iron temperature at 350° F or less.

2 Schedule regular trims. Get your relaxed ends cut off gradually and give yourself time to adjust to each new length.

3 Careful product application will help your new growth blend with your chemically-treated hair. Start at the roots (where you will need the most product) and work toward the ends.

Weekly Routine for Growing Out a Relaxer

Products & Tools Required

Shampoo

Deep Treatment

Leave-In Conditioner

Wide Tooth Comb

Rollers and/or Bobby Pins

Bonnet Dryer or Blow Dryer and Diffuser

Satin Scarf

Leave-In Products to Try

- ApHogee Gloss Therapy Polisher Spray
- As I Am Moisture Milk Daily Hair Revitalizer
- John Frieda Frizz-Ease Hair Serum, Thermal Protection Formula
- Nothing But Curl Sealer
- Silk Elements ColorCare Shine Spray

Step-By-Steps

Little details make a big difference! The step-by-step
care and styling tutorials in this chapter will help you get
consistent results every time, whether your hair is
natural or relaxed.

Pre-Shampoo Oil Treatment Tutorial

Key Tips

- Only do an oil treatment if you plan to shampoo, not co-wash. Co-washing will leave too much residue on your strands.
- Detangle your oil-coated hair with your fingers before you shampoo.
- Pay special attention to the most breakage prone (shortest) areas of your hair.

Step 1: On wash day, divide your dry hair into 4-6 sections. Do not wet your hair first.

Step 2: Apply a heavy coating of coconut oil throughout each section. Pay special attention to the most breakage prone areas of your hair. Use about 4 tablespoons depending on your strand thickness and length.

Step 3: Cover with a plastic cap to keep the oil from dripping down your face and neck and wait 20 minutes to 1 hour. It is best to give the oil time to soak into the outer cuticle layer of your hair. If you are short on time, skip to step 4.

Step 4: Before you get in the shower, lightly comb out your hair with your fingers to remove any tangles or knots. If you notice breakage as you finger comb, save detangling for the shower.

How to Shampoo and Condition
Coils & Curls

Key Tips

- Start by rinsing your hair for about 3 minutes.
- Massage, do not scratch your scalp as you shampoo.
- Comb your hair from ends to roots after you apply the conditioner.

Shampoo

Step 1: Gently comb through your dry hair with your fingers. Apply oil or a serum to areas that are very tangled.

Step 2: Once in the shower, rinse your hair with warm water for about 3 minutes. This long rinse will loosen up and rinse away product build up from the week.

Step 3: Apply a quarter-sized amount of shampoo to your scalp and hair. Add more water to help you lather and distribute the shampoo.

Step 4: Gently rub your scalp with the shampoo lather. Don't scratch your scalp because you'll cause tiny cuts that could affect your hair growth.

Step 5: Gently and quickly, work shampoo through the length of your hair.

Step 6: Always fully rinse your hair before applying conditioner.

Condition

Step 1: Work a generous amount of conditioner through your hair from root to tip.

Step 2: Add more water to your hair to help you distribute the conditioner. Make sure every strand is saturated. Leave the conditioner in your hair for the amount of time specified in the instructions on the bottle. Only use heat if that is part of the instructions.

Step 3: Before you rinse out the conditioner, detangle your hair with a wide tooth comb. Remember to start combing at the ends and work your way to the roots.

Step 4: Rinse thoroughly.

Step 5: The next product you apply will depend on the style you are trying to achieve.

Co-Wash Tutorial

Co-washing means "washing" your hair with conditioner. It is a way to refresh your hair when you don't have time to do your full shampoo and condition routine.

Key Tips

- Start by rinsing your hair for about 3 minutes.

- Co-washing is not effective enough to be your only method of cleansing. Use shampoo to cleanse your hair and scalp at least once a week.

- If your scalp becomes flaky or itchy, co-washing is not a good cleansing method for your hair.

Step 1: Rinse your hair with warm water for about 3 minutes. This long rinse will loosen up dirt and residue, which is especially important since you won't be using shampoo.

Step 2: Apply a generous amount of conditioner to your hair.

Step 3: Gently massage your scalp and hair with the product. Add more water to your hair to create a creamy lather.

Step 4: Make sure you have added enough conditioner so that your hair is easy to comb. Use a wide tooth comb to detangle your hair so that it is smooth and tangle-free. Rinse thoroughly. If you see breakage as you comb, skip this step.

Step 5: Style your hair and allow it to air dry. There will still be product residue on your hair and it will cause your hair to burn from heat styling. Limit your use of heat to a blow dryer with a diffuser attachment or a bonnet dryer on Low.

No Frizz Twist-Out Tutorial

"Twist-outs" are the go-to choice for wet setting natural hair. This tutorial will allow you to transform your natural coils and curls into a fluffy wave pattern, no heat required.

Key Tips

- To elongate your curls and decrease drying time, wait until your hair is over 50% dry before you start twisting sections.

- Touch your hair as little as possible as you air dry.

- Use a shine or anti-frizz serum to smooth fly aways and avoid frizz.

Step 1: Shampoo and condition or co-wash your hair.

Step 2: Do not towel dry your hair. Towel drying will cause irreversible frizz. Drape a towel over your shoulders to catch the drips.

Step 3: Apply a thorough coating of leave-in conditioner or styling cream to your soaking wet hair.

Step 4: Comb the product through with a wide tooth. Be generous; it is better to use too much than too little. Apply extra product to your roots.

Step 5: Air dry for 30-45 minutes. You want your hair to be more damp than dry.

Step 6: Once your hair is just slightly damp, begin twisting it into 2-strand sections. Apply a small amount of a shine or anti-frizz serum to each section as you twist. Smaller sections (about ½ inch wide) are best for finer strands because they make a tighter wave pattern.

Step 7: For extra fullness, add a curler to the end of some or all of the twists. Use rollers with a diameter between ½ and 1 inch. If you are transitioning to natural, the rollers will help your straight ends blend with your new growth.

Step 8: It is best to air dry your hair from this point. Air-drying is always the healthiest option, but if you don't have the extra time, use a blow dryer with a diffuser attachment. 15-20 minutes on Low or Warm should be enough to fully set your hair.

Step 9: Once your hair is completely dry, rub a small amount of serum through your hands. Use your serum-coated fingers to unravel each twist. Separate and fluff the areas of your hair where you want to create volume. Focus on the hair closer to your roots so you don't lose curl definition at your ends.

Step 10: Don't try to fluff your curls to perfection. As always, the less you touch your hair the better. Instead, leave some areas "piecey" and "un-fluffed". As you finish getting ready, your curls will naturally fall into place.

Step 11: At night, re-twist your hair into a few big sections and cover with a satin scarf.

How to Safely Straighten Relaxed Hair

Key Tips

- Avoid putting any heat on your hair unless it has been freshly shampooed and conditioned.

- To air dry with smooth results, apply a heat protection serum or foam immediately after towel-blotting your hair

- Make sure your flat iron has an LCD temperature control, so you can use minimal heat.

Step 1: Shampoo and deep condition your hair.

Step 2: Comb a heat protection serum or foam through with a wide tooth comb.

Step 3: Air dry without touching your hair until it is no longer damp. Check the roots to be sure. Air-drying is the healthiest option for relaxed hair.

Step 4: Add polish and movement with a ceramic flat iron. You will have to determine the amount of heat that is best for your hair, but 300°F is a good starting point.

Step 6: Gather the majority of your hair into 3 to 5 jaw clips, leaving a small section down in the very back. Make a horizontal part across the back of your head, near the base of your neck so you can straighten one row at a time.

Step 7: Flat iron 1-inch wide sections working from left to right and bottom to top. Use just enough heat that you only need 1 or 2 passes per section.

Step 8: Finish the style by applying a small amount of shine serum to smooth any fly aways.

Step 9: At night, wrap, pin curl, or braid your hair and cover it with a satin scarf.

How to Protect Your Hair While Swimming

Key Tips

- If possible, rinse your hair with tap water before you get in the pool.

- Don't wear a swim cap if it pulls too tightly or rips out your hair at the hairline.

- Always shampoo after you swim, chlorine does not rinse out.

Step 1: If possible, rinse your hair in the shower before getting in the pool. If your hair is "filled up" with tap water, it won't be able to absorb as much chlorinated pool water.

Step 2: Apply a generous coating of a hair serum to your dripping wet hair, paying special attention to the ends. The serum will help protect your hair from friction as you swim.

Step 3 (Optional): Put on a swim cap. Many swim caps are so tight that they pull your hair out when you take them off. If a swim cap causes you to lose hair, don't use it. Just let your strands hang free instead.

Step 4: After you swim, rinse your hair with tap water as soon as possible even if you're not ready to shampoo. It is best to wear a hat if you plan to stay in the sun after you get out of the pool.

Step 5: Always shampoo your hair after you are done swimming for the day. It is important to use a shampoo that gets rid of chlorine and mineral residue. If your regular shampoo contains chelating ingredients like Disodium EDTA or Phytic Acid it should be able to remove chlorine. If your regular shampoo does not contain EDTA or Phytic Acid, try using Ultra Swim Chlorine Removal Shampoo on pool days.

Step 6: Continue with your usual wash day routine. You must take the time to condition your hair every time you shampoo it, even if you swim every day.

Step 7: when you style your hair, it would be best to avoid direct or high heat. Try to limit your use of heat to a blow dryer with a diffuser attachment or a bonnet dryer on Low.

Thank You

I sincerely thank you for purchasing Coils & Curls The Hair Product Handbook. I set out to write an easy-to-follow guide that would truly change your hair life and I hope I have accomplished that. You can get started with a new routine today by checking the products in your stash against the lists in Chapter 3. After that, you can visit HairLiberty.org for style ideas, tutorials, and more about hair science. Remember, your hair can make you feel beautiful and confident or overwhelmed and frustrated...the right products and techniques make all the difference.

Made in the USA
Lexington, KY
12 January 2014